Aging Through a Pandemic

The Impact of COVID-19 on Ontarian Seniors

Viveka Sainani | Shirley Liu | Nancy Liu

Copyright © 2021
Viveka Sainani, Shirley Liu, Nancy Liu
All rights reserved.

No part of this publication may be reproduced, distributed, or transmitted in any forms or by any means, including photocopying, recording, or other electronic or mechanical method, without the prior written permission of the authors, except in the case of brief quotations embodied in critical reviews and certain other non-commercial uses permitted by copyright law.

First edition September 2021

Cover design by Disha Rawal

ISBN 979-8-4772-9564-7 (paperback)

Disclaimer

Although the authors have made every effort to ensure that the information in this book was correct at press time, the authors do not assume and hereby disclaim any liability to any party for any loss, damage, or disruption caused by errors or omissions, whether such errors or omissions result from negligence, accident, or any other cause.

CONTENTS

PREFACE	i
INTRODUCTION	iii
CHAPTER 1	
I. Michelle	1
II. Janet	5
III. Sean	7
IV. Stephanie	9
V. Chris	13
VI. Emily	15
VII. Eric	18
VIII. Megan	20
IX. Henry	23
X. Matilda	26
XI. Sophie	28
XII. Andrew & Fiona	30
CHAPTER 2	
I. The Importance of Support Systems	34
II. The Ups and Downs of the Media	36
III. The Impact of Technology During the Pandemic	38
IV. Challenges in Nursing and Long-Term Care Homes	41
V. Persistence Through Teamwork, Patience, and Positivity	43
BIBLIOGRAPHY	45
ACKNOWLEDGEMENTS	47
ABOUT THE AUTHORS	48

PREFACE

    Since the early spring of 2020, the COVID-19 pandemic has swept across the globe and caused drastic changes to the lives of billions of people. The elderly were one of the most vulnerable populations struck by this deadly disease, with the virus spreading rapidly through long-term care homes and retirement residences. It was devastating to the individual families and our community as a whole each time that we lost an elderly member. Now over a year into the pandemic, widespread vaccination and the development of preventative measures has helped contribute to the control of the COVID-19 outbreak in these residences. We turned to seniors in Ontario to listen to their experiences through these past years and the impact the pandemic has had on their lives. Through our interviews, we aim to preserve their stories and the struggles they have gone through during the pandemic. We hope this book can serve as a time-capsule of the pandemic as well as a stepping stone to building a better future that provides for our at-risk populations.

INTRODUCTION

COVID-19 is an infectious disease caused by the SARS-CoV-2 virus, first identified in December 2019 in Wuhan, China. The Chinese government rapidly responded by imposing strict travel bans and lockdowns, implementing mandatory city-wide screening, and constructing specialized testing centers and hospitals (Cyranoski, 2020; Cheng et al., 2020; Dong, 2021). While the outbreak was largely under control in China after two months of lockdown, the highly infectious virus had already spread to other continents. On January 25, 2020, Canada's "Patient Zero" - the first COVID-19 case in the country - was identified in Toronto (Staff, 2020). Since then, a combination of factors such as the delay in government response, reluctancy and misinformation to the public health guidelines and vaccine hesitancy, cycles of early community re-openings and the emergence of more infectious variants, have resulted in an inability to fully control the pandemic (Robertson, 2021). As of September 2021, Canada has tallied over 1.5 million COVID-19 cases and 27 000 deaths (Government of Canada, 2021).

One of the hardest-hit populations in Canada were the elderly living in retirement residences and long-term care homes. These people are at higher risk of infection and death from COVID-19 due to their age, comorbid medical conditions, and tight living spaces in these facilities. Over 80% of reported COVID-19 deaths during the first pandemic wave in Canada (March through August 2020) were of residents in long-term care homes (CIHI, 2020). The disproportionate incidence of COVID-19 infections in these homes has been attributed to staff shortage, lack of personal protective equipment (PPE), limited testing capacity, and close contact between residents and staff (Vilches et al., 2020). The pandemic has also had a negative impact on the mental well-being of seniors. Social isolation, loneliness, and the loss of loved ones contributed to increased depression and anxiety in older adults also in the United States amid the COVID-19 pandemic (Koma et al., 2020).

In order to preserve the stories of Ontarian seniors through the COVID-19 pandemic, we searched for seniors aged 65+ in Ontario who were willing to be interviewed over the phone for approximately one hour to share their stories. We spoke to 5 seniors from a retirement residence, 1 senior from a long-term care home accompanied by his wife, and 10 seniors living in their own homes. We achieved verbal or written consent from each interviewee prior to each interview. Additionally, we provided mental health resources in case of any discomfort and distress in remembering past experiences. Writing this book was truly a pleasure, and we are immensely grateful to our interviewees for sharing their experiences, thoughts and advice during the pandemic.

Our book is divided into two chapters. The first chapter compiles the stories of our interviewees, beginning with their pseudonym, each individual's background and transitioning into their experiences during the pandemic. We end each story with words of advice they have for the younger generation in regard to handling the pandemic and other times of difficulty. In the second chapter, we analyze the stories and highlight common themes among them. We then expand on each theme and offer our own insights.

We hope that through this book, readers from a wide range of ages and backgrounds will have something worthwhile to gain from our elders. For those who seldom speak to the seniors of their community, we see this as a useful medium for achieving a better understanding and appreciation of their experiences. Although we are all facing our own difficulties during the pandemic, it is important to not forget the individuals who have lived through so much yet are the most vulnerable to the deadly disease. There is still much more for us to learn and more work to be done in supporting the growing aging population. The first step is to listen with compassion and open hearts, and we believe this is a valuable place to start.

Chapter 1

I. Michelle

"Everyone is fighting a hard battle"

Early life:
    Michelle is 69 years old. She grew up in Southwestern Ontario in a large family of seven children, so she was accustomed to having a lifestyle surrounded by people and being constantly on-the-go. As one of the older children, she often found her hands full of responsibilities, albeit difficult to manage at times. She remembers biking to the bank with her dad's paycheck when she was only 10 years old, alongside other responsibilities like doing the dishes and laundry and looking over her younger siblings. Due to growing up in a large family, loneliness is now strongly felt when she's by herself.
    Michelle grew up not having a set path in mind, which enabled her to explore new things with freedom and curiosity. She attended university for one year to see if teaching was a possible career, but soon realized it was not for her. She found her passion when she crossed into the field of healthcare, where she worked as a medical lab technologist for 40 years. She loved her career; she always had the opportunity to try many different things and take on new challenges. From working in the blood bank, to hematology, to the core lab, she loved learning how to use new machines and administer new tests. For her, the endless opportunities to acquire new skills

was one of the most enticing and memorable parts of her career.

Retirement:

Although Michelle felt very passionately about her job, shift work was difficult and physically taxing. Fatigue became a larger issue as she grew older, and she retired at the age of 60. She and her husband Sam sold their house and put some money aside in case they needed long-term care later on, but they first moved into a retirement residence. Since then her life slowed down, and she had the opportunity to meet many new friends from the retirement home.

However, with a new segment of her life also came new challenges. Her husband was diagnosed with dementia. Michelle tried to remain calm and not let her fears and worries get in the way. To educate herself on how to better care for her husband, she took a course on dementia through McCormick Home, a not-for-profit long-term care facility. One of the most challenging aspects was dealing with Sam's denial that he suffered from this disease. She describes him as very stubborn and strong-willed - he wasn't very receptive to her taking the dementia course, so she had to sit on the porch with her earphones in order to listen to the classes. Overcoming the initial denial was a major hurdle, but Michelle was fortunate to have friends in the community to support her, as well as a social worker and nurse. Moreover, she saw this as an opportunity to continue her passion for life-long learning. With her new knowledge and experience dealing with dementia, she was now able to lend a hand to others around her suffering from the same disease.

Life during the pandemic:

When the pandemic hit in 2020, Michelle was presented with yet another challenge: loneliness. She suddenly lost the activities that kept her spirit high: meeting outside with friends, having picnics, going to the mall. One of her favourite times was coffee hour on Thursday mornings, where there would be music, and speakers would come in to talk about topics like driving for seniors, osteoporosis, and memory-related diseases. She loved chatting with friends and being able to learn something new every week. With her regular lifestyle disrupted, social isolation was a new problem she had to overcome. Her son and daughter were out of town, and both were very busy with their own lives and were unable to give much support. Furthermore, their generational gap made it sometimes difficult to relate to one another. For example, her children would keep telling her to buy groceries online, but Michelle was already accustomed to shopping in person and picking out her own food. For her, such a dramatic change in lifestyle is not as easy as it may sound to the younger generation.

Michelle relied on other seniors in her building for a sense of community during that time, and at the same time she reached out and helped others feel at home. She established a weekly habit of making 15–20-minute calls to seniors who were also isolated and didn't have family in town. Most of the seniors in the building received the support they needed. For those without family nearby or with serious illnesses, the church stepped in to help deliver groceries.

To cope with the changes caused by the pandemic, Michelle put structure into her days. She would walk early in the morning, spend some time in the exercise room with the bike, make meals with her husband, and watch some news on the TV. She also occupied herself by finding projects that gave her joy. For example, she took part in a project in her community where she made cards for other seniors living in long-term care homes. As a hands-on person, Michelle also found joy in making drapes for her husband's room.

Perhaps one of the most important factors in her ability to cope during the pandemic was the wonderful community she lived in. Everyone looked out for one another and always reached out with a kind heart. Those with cars unconditionally offered to drive others around if they needed to. Even a simple gesture like delivering papers to each other's doors was something that meant a lot. Michelle also recalls arriving at her front steps to see food hanging on her door. It was these simple acts of kindness that helped her overcome the most difficult moments of the pandemic.

Advice for the younger generation:
Now over a year into the pandemic, Michelle has had the opportunity to reflect about her lived experiences as a senior. She advises to learn to forgive people, and understand that everyone is going through something in life - "Don't be quick to judge and always leave your heart open."

She also wants others to know that there is a solution to every problem, even if it may seem like there isn't at the moment. Take every opportunity as a learning experience. She points to her husband's dementia again, and how through her love for learning she was able to take courses on how to care for those suffering from the disease. She encourages others to be a life-long learner and seek new challenges to overcome.

In regard to handling a pandemic, her advice is to just be patient and know that we will get to the other side. She understands younger people like fast solutions - just like the way they read text messages. As someone who still uses a flip phone, Michelle has grown used to not reading messages instantaneously. She knows there is a light at the end of the tunnel, but we must be patient and live one day at a time. Most importantly, give kindness to someone, and it will return.

II. Janet

"Have something planned and to look forward to"

Early life and retirement:
 Janet was born in London, Ontario as the tenth of eleven kids, and she has lived in this city her entire life. She got married at the age of 17 and had three children. She spent much of her life working in a medical clinic with two family doctors before she retired.
 Janet is now 69 years old and currently lives in a retirement residence. She found that life became much quieter when she became a senior as she lives by herself. Thankfully, she has made some connections with others living in her community, and they often meet up and have socials together. In her spare time, she keeps herself occupied by volunteering at a church and doing artwork such as painting and crafts.

Life during the pandemic:
 The liveliness of the community quickly turned into silence when the pandemic reached London. Everyone stayed home, and Janet, along with many other seniors, felt the days stretch long as she spent them alone. She recalled the moment when she retired and how excited she was to have no daily schedule. Now, during the pandemic, she realized how important it was to have something planned, something to look forward to. She even thought about

returning to her job and working part time to keep herself occupied. For her, one of the most dreadful parts of being in isolation was not knowing what day it was, as everything seemed to blend. She was no longer able to use her normal daily activities to break up her day.

Fortunately, she was still able to maintain some connection with her family and friends through Facetime and phone calls. Neither of her children live in the city, but they made attempts to talk to her every day and make sure everything was going well. She really appreciated having someone to talk to during these tough times. The church also called the group once a month to ask if anyone needed anything, which she thought was very kind as not everyone had close friends. She felt lucky that she still found a way to reach out to people, and that made time easier to pass.

Advice for the younger generation:

After enduring many months of hardship and isolation, Janet's advice for the younger generation is to keep pushing forward. "Tomorrow is another day. There will be a light, so don't get too bound into what's happening at the time." Knowing that there is hope helped her cope with the dreadful long days. She has been resilient by pulling herself out of the agony of isolation and continuing to be positive, passing this light onto the next generation. She expresses the importance of maintaining a social support system and advises everyone to keep family close.

III. Sean

"Live your life the best you can with what you're given"

Early life and retirement:
    Sean is now 79 years old and lives in a retirement residence in Southwestern Ontario. He grew up in a small town and in a low-income family. He recalls that in his younger days, his biggest goal in life was "simply to survive". Fortunately, he was able to find a job in the plumbing industry, working as an Ontario sales manager for a large plumbing corporation. He loved the work he did and spent 40 years in the industry. He also got married and now has two wonderful grandchildren he often spends time around.
    When asked how his life changed when he retired, he says, "Not really - age is just a number. I just continued what I did before retirement, with more time to do what I wanted to do." He enjoys playing golf and going fishing, occasionally taking his two grandchildren with him.

Life during the pandemic:
    When the pandemic hit, Sean found the most challenging aspect was not being able to see his family as often. He missed having dinner with his son and two grandkids, and attending special events and celebrations. Nevertheless, he felt he received enough support during the pandemic; his son and grandsons were both in town and

were able to give weekly visits and frequent phone calls. When his family was not around, Sean reached out to other seniors in his residence, with whom he would go for walks in the area. Having a physically close support system was vital to preventing social isolation during the pandemic.

However, as Sean gained more awareness of the outside world through the media, he sometimes found himself crippled with anxiety. "There was so much negativity out there, and you just had to learn to turn it off." He reached out to his family doctor and started taking some anxiety medications. But with these medications also came side effects like vision and hearing problems, and more severe withdrawal. They affected him for about a month, but thankfully he has successfully recovered.

Advice for the younger generation:

When asked for words of advice for the younger generation in regard to handling unprecedented events like the pandemic, Sean says to "understand how easily everything can be upset in a hurry - sometimes you don't have any control on what happens, it's being done for you and against you. But live your life the best you can with what you're given, and don't take any days for granted."

Sean says the same advice can be applied to matters in everyday life. He believes the world is going too fast compared to 70 years ago. It's important to stop and take a minute to enjoy what you have, and know that not everything will be sunshine and roses. Having grown up in a low-income family, Sean feels his experience of working through having nothing, and getting to where he is has allowed him to open his vision on how the world works. He encourages the younger generation to take more time to explore the world and acquire new knowledge and skills. He jokes, "If you take 10 of the smartest people now, and throw them into the woods in Algonquin Park, they wouldn't know how to get out." Sean believes the younger generation depends too much on technology, and he hopes that we can look to the elderly to learn back the basic skills that have sustained us until today.

IV. Stephanie

"The jack of all trades, ace of none"

Early life:

Stephanie is an 84 year old who grew up in Guyana and moved to Canada after her husband came to Western University to become a professor. Most of her early life in Guyana was spent doing things she enjoyed, such as singing and dancing. After school, she would learn to knit, sew and crochet from her neighbour. After working in schools for a bit, her passion for working with kids pushed her to continue onto college for additional training in education. Stephanie loved to be involved and joined clubs for singing, poetry and drama during her college years. She reflected that she wasn't fully happy then because she was worried about passing her program at school. Although she made sure to make memories and enjoy along the way, she really maintained her focus on school.

During her time in college, her life took a dramatic turn. Her college was shut down because Guyana experienced a violent strike with people trying to burn down the capital. It was a terrible time for all students as they were unsure about their safety let alone if they could finish their education. Having lived through this, she learned to prioritise her professional goals and have faith in herself and others. She became resilient to change and always kept moving forward. As a teacher, Stephanie not only enjoyed teaching but also enjoyed the teachers' socials, dancing and excitement of life.

Stephanie met her husband at several meetings and conferences before getting married. Since he was a headmaster in a different city, she had to move to a more rural area with mainly rice farmers. She expressed how hard it was to leave the place where she had been born and bred. However, she also looked at the positives of her new life, noting "the farmers there always gave from their heart, sending me food or items, and I truly appreciate that they welcomed me with open arms". They occasionally took trips to visit relatives in other countries but most of her time off was spent sewing and enjoying time with her family. Her fondest memories of her married life were the time spent socializing with neighbours, family and friends. She talks about receiving help when adjusting to her new life and raising her two kids and says "one should always help people when you can, as a way to pay forward".

Stephanie continued to be resilient as she raised her kids alone for three years before she could join her husband in Canada. Eventually she made the move, starting as a student at Fanshawe college and continuing her studies at Western University. Her husband got a job in Northwestern Ontario teaching and she continued to directly support the family while studying. These were definitely hard times for her. She left her kids with a sitter, but when she cancelled, Stephanie would have to take the kids on the bus with her to university. She would leave her kids with the cafeteria staff while she was at work. She worked tirelessly to support her family yet she still believes that "things weren't as bad as they are now [in the sense that] no one fought as much and there wasn't as much violence".

Her husband would come back for Christmas when possible and had many plans to spend more time with his kids. However, things changed when he developed heart problems, and Stephanie saved six weeks of vacation to take the kids to visit him. She is a very hardworking woman who understood these sacrifices as "just part of life". Unfortunately, his health continued to deteriorate. One night while the kids were asleep, policemen knocked on her door and explained that her husband had a heart attack while playing tennis and died. Stephanie was not only traumatized by the news, but she was also in shock about how to continue raising two young kids. Luckily, her family friend took care of their house and belongings up north while her brother-in-law and some friends helped with funeral arrangements. She was grateful to be surrounded with a community to help her through these tough times.

Retirement:
When the time came, her kids got married and moved away for work. She had seniority at her job and was in no fear of losing it, so she continued to work. There came a time when her kids explained that the company was trying to push her out and that it would be better to retire. Luckily, her pension was enough to live the simple life she enjoyed. Being a very social person, she was worried about adjusting to retirement. She slowly weaned herself into staying at home more and picked up a few new hobbies. She realized it was time to sell her house and she decided on a retirement living not far from her house. She could continue to live the life she did, going to the same events and clubs, and seeing the same friends.

Her life up until the pandemic continued along the same lines. She was very busy, always out meeting people and exchanging experiences. She is also very religious and would go to a variety of local churches and study groups - attending an event a day for many years! In her words, she is "intrigued by people, places and things" and, "wasn't going to sit, mope and cry!" As the girl who lived among the rice farmers in Guyana, she would sometimes feed the birds around the property and pick up garbage outside her house. She has always had a sense of humanity and wants to make the world a better place in whatever way she can.

Life during the pandemic:
During the pandemic, she started phoning people and singing happy birthday to them as a way of keeping busy and lifting spirits. She is fortunate to be able to cook and bake more, and she continues

to find joy in these little things. Initially, it was tough because her friends in the residence were not able to play games together. She formed a club to sit outside and play games. She considered the pandemic just another event in life and was able to adapt well to the changes that came along.

She recognizes that the pandemic was tougher for other people, especially during the winter when you can't go outside as much. She says that a main challenge was transportation since she would usually get rides with people in her community. She would try to take the bus but they were not on time, often early and hard to anticipate.

Advice for the younger generation:

Living through the hardships of her country's instability, moving across the globe, and supporting her children alone, she has learned to always keep it light and enjoy life for what it is. When asked about the pandemic, her answers were simple and she never expressed much difficulty with adjusting, as she likes to call herself "the jack of all trades, ace of none". With that mentality, she hopes that the younger generation is able to "be genuine, soft but truthful". She gives good reminders to think about tomorrow when going about today and encourages the youth to be positive and never give up.

V. Chris

"Building a community on unconditional kindness"

Early life and retirement:
Chris is 87 years old and was born and raised in Britain. He studied engineering, then moved to Canada at the age of 19. Adjusting to the new life here was difficult - he continuously faced issues with low pay, abuse in the workplace, and layoffs. However, Chris overcame each challenge with determination. According to him, "Things were tough, but you find anything to make ends meet. You might not find an ideal job, but you take what's available." With this persistence, Chris eventually landed a stable job in an engineering company where he stayed for 35 years. He loved working there, as he got along with everyone else and was able to move up a few ranks.

Chris got married and had three children. Unfortunately, his marriage wasn't smooth, and he divorced from his wife and lost his house. Shortly after, he retired at the age of 65, but he stayed with his company for another two years and found some temporary work. He then decided he wanted to try something different, so he packed his belongings again and moved into a retirement residence.

He feels this environment is much better as he is surrounded by people his age with whom he can get along with well. Chris also found many ways to keep himself occupied in this new setting. He joined the committee for his senior home, where he currently serves as Treasurer. By getting together with others and organizing events, he has made many new friends and has built a very strong support system.

Life during the pandemic:

When the pandemic hit, however, all these social activities were terminated. Chris felt the most challenging part of living during the pandemic as a senior was simply "finding something to do." Although he was isolated, he explored new ways to keep himself busy. He discovered a love for playing card games on the computer, reading online articles, and watching YouTube videos. He was also fortunate to be within walking distance of the grocery store, library, and fitness centre. He says he has never felt unsafe or worried while outside, particularly in his area, so he was able to carry out most daily tasks unaffected. Most importantly, he had people around him in the building whom he could trust. For example, one night he had slipped and fallen, but he was able to reach for the phone and call for help. Others within the building quickly arrived to his attention and helped bring him to the emergency department. With this close support system in place, Chris has always felt safe and reassured during the pandemic.

Advice for the younger generation:

Drawing on his experiences and hardships growing up in Britain, to finding a stable job in Canada, and building strong relationships with other seniors in his community, Chris has learned the importance of returning kindness to others. "You have to have your eyes open. If someone appears to need help, offer help. Be more outgoing and don't run away from things. If the weather's bad and you see someone with difficulty, or if someone needs a lightbulb changed, offer to help." He believes by linking hands and building a society in which you give kindness unconditionally, any setbacks can be easily overcome.

VI. Emily

"It is different, but doable"

Early life and retirement:

Emily moved to Southwestern Ontario when she was married and has been living here ever since. She is now 78 years old and lives in a retirement residence, where she looks after herself.

Early in her life, her first priority was her family and so she dedicated 15 years to taking care of her family at home. She eventually sought a job as an educational assistant, where she worked for around 20 years.

When Emily turned 65, she retired and lived alone in her house for a few years. After realizing that was not the lifestyle she wanted, she decided to sell her house and move into a retirement residence.

Emily is now a widow, and she has gotten used to being on her own. Her son runs his own business north of Toronto, and she is thankful that he is close to home. On the other hand, her daughter works in Saudi Arabia at the University of Science and Technology, and she is proud of her for her successes in life and for finding a job that she loves.

There are many other seniors in her neighbourhood, some much older and some younger. It took a while for her to get to know everyone and to feel at home, but now they have formed a close bond. She got involved in her community, not only by taking evening walks with her neighbours, but also by volunteering at her local church and joining a stitch group. Before the pandemic, she kept herself busy and never had to worry about not having things to do.

Life during the pandemic:

When the pandemic hit, Emily found that the biggest challenge was having the enjoyable parts of her life cut out in a flash. There were no more playing games, eating at restaurants, or holding celebrations. The sudden change in her lifestyle was definitely difficult to adjust to. Thankfully though, she wasn't hurt in any way. She calls it "different, but doable". Her friends kept her company by phoning her, and she began to read a lot more to pass the time. She bought several Christian and Amish books and finds the stories very rewarding to read. She also loves watching sports. Although there were no spectators allowed this year, she feels fortunate that she could still watch the Olympics on the television.

Emily is very understanding, and when asked whether there was more that could have been done to address the hardships she faced, she responded that it was "very difficult for anyone". The pandemic spread almost instantly, and in a short time it was already all over Canada. It was not an easy task to manage this, but she expresses the need for greater support for nursing home residents. She had heard of the difficulties they experienced, especially the struggles of isolation, and expressed how crucial it is for them to have more contact with their family. Resources should also be provided to nursing homes quickly to protect them from the virus. She cautions against the reopening of borders, especially with the emergence of new variants. She couldn't believe how fast the virus spread from overseas and realized the need to react quickly to protect our vulnerable populations.

Advice for the younger generation:

In regard to how the younger generation has addressed the pandemic, Emily has a few pieces of advice she would like to share. Firstly, one must be patient. She witnessed younger individuals doing things that they were asked not to do, such as gathering in large groups. She understands that it is difficult for the younger generation because of how they were brought up - things were always there for them, like the Internet, and they could do anything they wanted. However, she has learned from her many experiences that some things don't come instantly. One must learn to think about others and not just themselves. Only this way, can we bring an end to this pandemic sooner and return to the normal life that we now all value.

VII. Eric

"Listen to proper people giving proper advice"

Early life and retirement:

Eric is a 70 year old senior who was born in Toronto, and he has lived in Canada his whole life. He used to work in Toronto where he drove streetcars, and later in life he moved to a suburban area in Southwestern Ontario. He currently lives in his own home, where his wife and two pet birds keep him company. He also collects Christmas albums as a hobby (he has over 200 of them!).

Unfortunately, due to increasing back pain, Eric decided to retire early. He has been trying to take care of his health since, but the condition has prevented him from doing many things he used to do. Now, at home he spends his days playing his favourite computer games and organizing his record collection in the basement. For most of the day, however, he rests on the couch to cope with his back pain.

Life during the pandemic:

Luckily, Eric expressed that the pandemic hasn't bothered him too much. He and his wife are "best friends", and they pass the time together by reading and watching TV. He does feel confined at times as he is unable to see his friends, but thankfully they are able to maintain contact by calling each other frequently. He has found it difficult to get support from others in his community, as everyone has their own problems to deal with. His back pain also became a bigger challenge as he could not get the medical attention he normally received. The pandemic made it much harder to book appointments with family physicians, let alone a specialist. At the end of the day, he is very appreciative of his wife as he relies on his wife the most for support.

Advice for the younger generation:

In regard to handling a crisis like the pandemic, Eric advises the younger generation to "listen to proper people giving proper advice". We must follow public health guidelines, even if it means sacrificing elements of our everyday lifestyle. Be tolerant, and be thoughtful of others. Everyone is in the same boat, and some might be in an even worse situation than you. The elderly population has it especially hard as they must manage health issues along with the pandemic, and this is something the younger generation often forgets. During times when everyone is facing hardship, mutual support is what is most needed. Intergenerational help would be beneficial to both the elderly and younger population as there is much to learn from each other.

VIII. Megan

"All it takes is one missed precaution"

Early life and retirement:
Megan was born in Belarus and moved to Canada at age 8. She is now 79 years old and has lived in the same city since. She lived a quaint life with her husband, their three kids and now has many grandchildren and great grandchildren. Megan tells us how fortunate she is to be close to her family and enjoy their company and support. When her husband passed away, she kept working without stopping to take a break and enjoy life. After retirement, she learned that the most important thing is to spend time with loved ones and enjoy every day.

Life during the pandemic:
Her typical day before the pandemic included reading, seeing her family and going to the movies. She has a boyfriend who lives about an hour away so she visits him when she can. Megan explains that the time during the pandemic was especially hard for her because both her brother and boyfriend have been diagnosed with cancer. This hits close to home as her husband lost his battle with cancer many years ago. The pandemic was a very stressful time for her and she often became very lonely not being able to go about her regular activities. She was thankful to have her granddaughter living close by

and was able to form a bubble with her. Though she tries to video chat with her other kids often, she struggles with watching her grandkids grow up from afar. She is saddened that she isn't able to spend time getting close with them.

Megan thoroughly expressed the importance of being cautious during the pandemic and that this must come before any longing for loved ones. During the height of the pandemic, her boyfriend would visit her when coming to her city for his cancer treatments. She was afraid to pass anything along to him, so she always wore a mask and emphasized its value. After a particular visit, she returned home and found out a week later that her boyfriend had COVID-19. She got tested immediately and was relieved that the result was negative. She says that without her mask, the virus would have spread so easily and that "all it would take was one day of skipping the regular precautions". Megan advises the youth to wear a mask, sanitize and stay inside when possible. She sacrificed a lot in order to stay safe and prevent the spread of the virus to others.

Megan had to have two surgeries during the pandemic and was surprised that some people in the hospital rooms didn't wear a mask. She was scared of such conditions and even wore a mask when sleeping because she would rather be safe than sorry. She believes that health care workers and teachers should be required to get vaccinated and that some employers should also consider this. Megan says that even though she was sick for five weeks after her vaccine, she still believes in its value and this is a testament to the importance of being vaccinated. She gave the example of kids not being able to bring peanut butter in schools because it could harm those with allergies. This is the same idea as being vaccinated to prevent others, who may not be able to get the vaccine, from contracting the virus.

Advice for the younger generation:
She truly believes that if everyone followed the rules and were cautious, the pandemic would have been over sooner. Both her daughter and granddaughter worked as waitresses during the

pandemic and they both have asthma. They had no issue wearing masks because they understood that not only their lives were at stake but also those around them. Being able to stay at home during the pandemic is a privilege not all of us have, so we should exercise that privilege to the best of our abilities. Those who must continue to work should be careful to follow guidelines as much as possible and understand that their sacrifice isn't going unnoticed.

IX: Henry

"Follow your heart and embrace change"

Early life:
   Henry is 81 years old and was born in New Hampshire. He grew up where there were mainly white French Canadian Catholics who worked in the textile and shoe mills. The diversity was sparse - he only knew of one Anglican church (but no one he knew attended) and only one black family in the community. He was a good student in high school and continued on to pharmacy school where he worked hard to complete his program. Henry met his wife in pharmacy school and was set to graduate when he received a government letter saying that he would have to attend military training. This was during the Vietnam war and as he was of age to join combat, he was worried that he might not graduate nor be able to continue. Luckily, he was one of 15 accepted to a hospital pharmacy internship program and was able to forgo military training to continue his education.
   Once he finished his internship, he got a job in a public health hospital in Maryland but soon he was offered a job on an Anishinaabe reserve in Minnesota. He had two children in Minnesota and spent lots of time fishing and hunting with the natives. Henry really enjoyed his time working at the reserve and expressed that "they are good people". He tells the story of sending

a patient to Minneapolis for a treatment. They came back without having gone to the appointment. When asked what happened, the patient explained that once he landed, he saw a friend that he hadn't met for years. He decided that the time spent with him was more valuable. Henry highlights that for Indigenous people, "time does not mean anything to them and they simply run on life". It was important to understand and acknowledge these differences.

Work life:

His work as a hospital pharmacist made him realize that he loved working in hospitals, so he went back to school to be able to work as a clinical pharmacist. After his education and training, he received a job offer in Boston and moved there. When he arrived, however, his employer informed him that the government denied the funding to supply his job. Henry was struck with the panic of losing his job alongside the stress of having to provide for his two children, wife, and another child soon to come. Luckily, there happened to be an executive leaving their post, so he was able to take over that job.

Henry lived through both the highs and lows of life and went along for the ride. At this point, he was commuting to Boston from New Hampshire and saw discrimination first hand. He was happy to see that a black woman had worked her way up the ranks in his facility. Though, he was sad that she wasn't as welcomed as he was. He says, "they called her an 'oreo', they said she was black on the outside and white on the inside". He insinuates that they discriminated against her based on how she was raised while he didn't get the same judgement since he was 'an outsider'.

Soon after, he got a job building community health centers in Canada and made the move across the border. He moved around a bit in Canada, as an executive director of many hospitals but he eventually retired in Southwestern Ontario. As a senior, he says he adjusted well. Throughout his travels, he always enjoyed the place for what it was and as he said, "I never looked back, always forward - appreciating the experience while I could".

Life during the pandemic:

During the pandemic, he says that he had no problems getting the essentials since he and his wife are not big shoppers. Having seen the rapid spread of COVID-19 throughout long-term care and nursing homes, he prefers living in his house for as long as possible. Being a public health expert, he believes that developing home health care services is the key to improvement in this area. Henry explains that retirement and long-term care homes can be expensive and that if you have assets you have to pay more. Additionally, there are very few service hours a month and that living in a small apartment with a few in-home health services could be a much better option.

Advice for the younger generation:

Reflecting on his life, Henry advises the younger generation to study something passionately but also understand that you might want something different later on in life. When this happens, don't be afraid to follow your heart and embrace change. This is true not only in life but specifically for the pandemic. These drastic changes should be taken in stride. Understanding that everything in life is an experience to be had and that this moment will never come back is crucial to seeing the silver lining and to keep moving forward in life!

X: Matilda

"Extra long, dark nights will end"

Background:
Matilda was born in New Delhi, India. She came to Canada when she was 26 years old, where she completed a postdoctoral fellowship. She is now 87 years old and living at home alone. Matilda is an independent person who manages well by herself. She enjoys going out and interacting with others through activities such as exercise classes, book clubs, and outdoor events.

Life during the pandemic:
As many activities were canceled due to the pandemic, Matilda was emotionally affected as she felt there were no more special occasions in her daily life. She struggled to feel like she was starting a new day as each one blended into the next. She described feeling like the pandemic was "one long period of time". She slowly learned to accept her new unusual lifestyle but is looking forward to activities opening up soon and resuming her fulfilling life.

Despite the difficulties she faced, she was thankful she was offered help by many people. Her friends supported her not only by doing her shopping but also helping in simple ways like talking to her when she was lonely. These interactions have taught her the importance of kindness during challenging times like the pandemic.

Her story highlights the contributions a social support system can have on the elderly living in a pandemic.

Advice for the younger generation:

To the younger generation, Matilda wishes that they pass each day one at a time, accept the circumstances, and obey the rules. It is not the end of the world! She has endured many other manmade and natural disasters such as war and famines, and she has learned that "extra long dark nights will end". With her strength and persistence, she has been able to withstand the many struggles throughout her 87 years. She encourages the younger generation to do the same - we must hang tight, stay optimistic, and assure ourselves that we can overcome this pandemic.

XI. Sophie

"A flame of hope through it all"

Early life and retirement:

Sophie is 84 years old and grew up in France. She moved to Canada after meeting a Canadian soldier in the air force, where she married him and had two kids. She has now lived in Canada for over 50 years. She came from a big family of 20 children, but there are now only one of her siblings left. Sadly, one of her children also passed away a few years ago. Having lost so many people in her life, she explains that "you just keep coping", but both her and her husband's health hasn't been the same since the passing of their child.

Life during the pandemic:

Before the pandemic, Sophie and her husband would enjoy camping and boating as well as spending time with their kids and grandkids. Since their decline in health, travel has been more difficult. As an elder, shopping with too many people was also a challenge. Despite all this, she says the biggest challenge of the pandemic is not being able to see the people you want to see. She understands that many people get agitated and more anxious during a time like this. She hopes that everyone takes the right measures but she understands that there is still fear because you never really know if you're safe.

She loves the French countryside and misses visiting her family in France. She hasn't been back for 21 years and wishes she could have visited more often before the pandemic. Sophia is fortunate that she still has her mother who was able to come visit her four times this year. She struggles to maintain her health while caring for her husband but was relieved to have her mother's support during this tough time.

Sophie copes as best she can but sometimes must put the needs of her loved ones above her own. She was set to get surgery on her foot but she hasn't been able to have the procedure since her husband's diagnosis with bone cancer. She shared the difficulty of the situation as her husband had prostate cancer before and is fighting cancer once again. Sophie knows that prolonging her surgery puts her at risk of not being able to walk and that this might be a reality very soon. However, she can't bear to leave her husband's side and doesn't even think about herself right now. Sophie is a flame of hope, being so strong while managing through all these difficult events.

Advice for the younger generation:

Sophie hopes that humanity is back on its feet soon and that people get vaccinated as it's been a long and hard pandemic for many people. She is sad to see so many people pass away but is very happy to hear when younger people choose to get vaccinated. She advises the youth to think about others as there are hidden struggles in every generation, and she hopes that we can all help each other when possible.

XII. Fiona & Andrew

"Listen to every voice at the table"

Early life and retirement:
Fiona is 75 years old and has been living alone for about three years since her husband, Andrew, moved into a long-term care home. They are both from India but met in England where he was a doctor and she was a nurse before coming to Canada. They have lived in Canada for 46 years and have raised one daughter.

At first, Andrew wanted to study engineering but as his schooling went on, he became very interested in nutrition and decided to pursue medicine. Fiona explained that throughout his life, he really loved to help people, especially in a hospital setting. He served as a role model for students and helped pave the path for others. When he came to Canada, he redid his medical education. During his residency, he realized his true passion was in pathology.

When he retired, he was able to focus more specifically on being a nutritionist. He opened a practice to help people with their diet. Before retirement, Fiona and Andrew travelled yearly but after retirement, they travelled less because of their nutrition practice and many social events with friends. He was always someone who took good care of his health and stayed active with his hobbies such as golf and badminton. Unfortunately, within the last couple of years, he developed shingles and then soon after, he was diagnosed with

Parkinson's disease. To receive the support he needs he moved into a long-term care home, where he currently resides. Even in the face of hardships arising from his own health, his wife mentions that he was always grounded and kind, trying to help people whenever he could. When he joined the long-term care home, Fiona would visit him every day and take him to the coffee shop downstairs to spend time and have a change of scenery. They are each other's main support system.

Life during the pandemic:

When the pandemic struck, she was not able to visit him which was very isolating for both of them. As the homes slowly adapted to the pandemic, Andrew was allowed one caregiver to visit initially, and now two to three visitors accompanied by a caregiver. Now, Fiona visits him once a week and also stays in touch with him through Facetime calls arranged by the staff. Fiona says, "the staff is quite supportive and careful about screening people before seeing patients. If anything happens while you're not there, they will always inform the family immediately about any changes with the patient."

With the pandemic also came changes in social life. Before the pandemic, staff would sometimes take the residents out to the bowling alley, but now they have activities within the home. Andrew coped by listening to spiritual music on his iPad, watching TV to keep himself informed about the world, and reading. The home kept him quite busy with a usual routine of breakfast at 8:30 am, some form of activity such as physio, gym, shower, mental games or quizzes and a snack before lunch. They would repeat a similar routine before dinner. Andrew is also very fortunate that his brother visits every other day to keep him company and have in-person interactions now that he is fully vaccinated.

Fiona explains that it was hard for her because she knows that if it were not for the pandemic, he would be able to come home to visit. She kept busy by calling friends who gave her the energy to keep going. However, she states that "when talking to upbeat friends on the phone, you can see that they too are not as upbeat and are more somber." She understands that collectively, everyone was dealing with something during the pandemic and it was hard to stay in touch with friends and family.

Advice for the younger generation:

Fiona emphasizes that you should never take anything for granted. Reflecting on her and Andrew's life, she says "try to do as much as you can in your early life because you don't know what will happen later, take everyday seriously but no play isn't good either." As a nurse, she understands that sometimes people think they know better than others, and this results in some people's voices getting overshadowed. She says to always listen to what others have to say because each person has gone through a lot in their life. She believes you can learn many things from listening to everyone and where they are coming from. It might only be in the long term that you understand what they were saying is true, so it is better to consider everything properly first. Reflecting on Andrew's life, she says to always help whoever you can along the way, have friends and hobbies, and take every minute of your day seriously because life is valuable.

Chapter 2

I. The Importance of Support Systems

For many of the seniors, the greatest challenge brought on by the pandemic was social isolation. Especially for retired individuals who spend much of their time outside and socializing with others, the dramatic shift to staying at home was a difficult adjustment to make. Throughout the interviewees' stories, it is evident that a close support system is critical for helping them cope with loneliness. Unfortunately, not all of them had family close by, and those who did were very extremely grateful for it. Sean expressed how lucky he felt that his sons and grandsons were in the same city and were able to give him weekly visits. For Sophie, while most of her family is in France, her mother visited her several times this year and helped her feel more at home. Eric mentioned how his wife is his greatest support system, being his "best friend" and spending every day with him.

Those who could not directly contact their family received support in other ways. Almost all of them mentioned having regular phone calls or video chats, either with friends or family. We saw that some elders were able to modify their social groups to maintain some level of support, such as Stephanie calling friends to wish them happy birthday or Megan forming a social circle with her son and grand-daughter. Reaching out to friends was a great solution but in Fiona's case, she still felt that it wasn't enough because her outgoing and energetic friends were equally dealing with their own dramatic shifts. Other individuals were also fortunate to receive support from their local church, who made frequent phone calls to ask if everything was alright or helped deliver groceries. Driving and shopping for one another were a few other good deeds that the seniors, like Michelle, were thankful for. Even in times of emergency, there were people available to help. For example, Chris gave the frightening example of when he suffered a fall in his home, but fortunately he was able to call for help and get others to send him to the Emergency Department. It is during situations like this that we truly appreciate the people we have around us and understand the importance of maintaining a close social network.

With the generous support that the seniors received, many of them also began to return the favour to others in need. Michelle described establishing a weekly habit of phoning other residents in her building who did not have family nearby. Stephanie, who always loved making the world a brighter place, formed a club of people from her residence to sit outside and play games. Here, we see the impact of mutually beneficial interactions as they help the entire community grow together during times of difficulty. Although this pandemic has taken away from our everyday lives, we also have the opportunity to give back to others and make someone else's day a little better.

II. The Ups and Downs of the Media

Many elderly people turned to the media as a way to educate themselves on current events in the world. Andrew started watching and reading the news while Chris turned to YouTube videos. Emily was grateful to be able to watch the Olympics on TV after in-person spectators were prohibited. While everyday life was on pause, the media enabled seniors to continue to immerse themselves in the world. They could stay in touch with what was happening and get in on the action in real-time.

While the media has its advantages, trying to be more plugged in and socially aware via the media can be difficult for a generation learning how to use it. Sean struggled with crippling anxiety as a result of gaining more awareness of the world around him through the media. As the pandemic reduced the number of activities possible and forced more people to stay at home, Sean went online and used the media as his main source of information. It is recognized that exposure to violent media is a major public health problem and that it is linked to anxiety in adolescents (Madan et al., 2013). Some youth however have become desensitized to the violence in the media given they have had more exposure to it. In contrast, the seniors are now turning to the media via online platforms to stay in touch with the world during the pandemic. The shift in the media to more negative news stories can come as a shock to those elderly that are not used to seeing simultaneous catastrophic events. Notable examples of these events that occurred during the pandemic include the terrorist attack on Muslims in London, Ontario, discovery of unmarked graves at residential schools in British Columbia, and the housing crisis nation-wide. We postulate that negative media during the pandemic, alongside social isolation, may have contributed to worsening of depressive symptoms and mood in seniors.

Growing up with social media, many of the youth are used to dealing with the negative effects of the media. Some still struggle with anxiety and depression and so it is hard to imagine the impact it has on the elderly. During the pandemic, the elderly who turned to technology to deal with social isolation may have become very aware of the many downsides of the media and see this contribute to a decline in their mental well-being. Using the media to learn about current issues can be helpful but Sean, like many other seniors, quickly saw that having a plethora of news at your fingertips can become overwhelming.

III. The Impact of Technology During the Pandemic

In Stephanie's story, we heard that she had to stop college due to an ongoing strike in her country. She was worried that she would lose a year of school. During Henry's time, he was hoping to be able to continue school instead of training for the military during the Vietnam war. Parallels can be drawn with students studying during the pandemic. Initially, there was talk of losing a year of school and worry that kids wouldn't graduate. School is a privilege and we are fortunate that there has been so much progress in technology to be able to have online school. As university students, we are lucky that our education could continue online as that wasn't a possibility previously.

Most of the past pandemics took place before the . According to the US Public Health report following the 1918–1919 Spanish flu, many schools shut down because they could not maintain proper sanitation (Stern et al., 2010). If this were the current situation, schools would have been closed without any hope of continuing or would have remained open with a much higher rate of infection. Our advances in technology since then have increased communication across the world. People can not only stay in touch with their loved ones but globally, countries are able to communicate quickly and effectively. This enables the rapid distribution of personal protective equipment (PPE), vaccines and other resources to continue life in the well known 'new normal'.

Seeing advancement and implementation of technology into everyday life has facilitated global communication as well as the transition to online learning and remote work. However, many seniors still expressed difficulty in adapting to the use of technology throughout the pandemic. For example, Michelle pointed out that while her children simply ordered groceries online, she preferred going to grocery stores in person to pick out her own food. She says that when you have spent your entire life living one way, it is extremely difficult adjusting to change, especially when you are not living in close proximity to younger people. As we've all realized throughout the pandemic, interacting through technology is very different from in-person interactions. Fiona found that her energetic friends, that kept her going, couldn't give her that same energy over the phone. She attributes this to everyone's subdued mood during the pandemic but there is also the added element of the medium. Meanwhile, youths who have grown up communicating via text messages experienced a relatively easier transition to pandemic life. The discordance in the way we utilize technology, has further contributed to the generational gap between youths and seniors. While seniors struggle to understand life online, youth can be oblivious to life in-person.

Some say that the youth have gone too far integrating in-person life and technology. Sean feels strongly about how technology has affected the younger generation. He believes youths are too attached to technology and this has resulted in a lack of understanding of how the world works. While a smartphone can provide so many functions and help us become more efficient in daily tasks, he says we have lost fundamental knowledge that everyone in his generation had. His example of taking 10 of the smartest people now into Algonquin Park to see who would be able to get out is a great highlight of the kinds of life skills that he believes many people lack today. He hopes the younger generation can take more time to go out into the world, explore, and learn how everything works.

The analogy Sean made can also be applied to the way younger people have responded to the pandemic. When communities first shut down, there was an overwhelming wave of panic, particularly in the younger generation. Many people have developed a lifestyle of going out for meals, such that they have lost the basic ability to cook for themselves. Research suggests that since the mid-1900s, Americans have shown a decline in consumption from home food sources and the amount of time spent cooking at home (Smith et al., 2013). Although lockdowns have given people more time to explore and develop cooking skills, a survey shows that consumers are getting increasingly tired of eating from home (Devenyns, 2020). It is evident how important a role restaurants play in our society now - every time restrictions are lifted, one of the first places to be filled with people are diners. Hopefully, the pandemic has allowed the younger generation to realize the importance of such basic life skills, and to take more time to develop them so they can better sustain themselves during times of hardship like the pandemic.

There are many lessons to be learned from the pandemic. The youth are fortunate to be able to continue school online as is everyone working from home. On a global scale, there is also a lot to appreciate but seniors continue to struggle with ever-changing technology. While seniors can learn from the youth, we see that the street goes both ways. The youth have much to learn from seniors and, as Michelle said when she took classes to educate herself on dementia, it is never too late to learn something new. We should all have an open vision, embrace the concept of life-long learning, and be curious about how the world works.

IV. Challenges in Nursing and Long-Term Care Homes

Many of our interviewees were living at home or in retirement residences. We saw that these individuals were able to manage well for the most part, as they stayed close to their loved ones and kept in touch with their peers. However, some individuals expressed that the situation was at an entirely different level for those living in nursing or long-term care homes. Emily was especially concerned about social isolation when these facilities prohibited visitors. Although she was able to maintain connections with friends and family through phone calls, she understands that this was much more difficult for nursing home residents who are physically incapable of doing so. Emily wishes that more could have been done to help residents keep in contact with family.

Another important area of concern that some interviewees addressed was the rapid spread of COVID-19 through nursing and long-term care homes. Henry lives in his own house, but after seeing the devastating effects of the virus in the facilities, he hopes to remain in his house for as long as possible. He emphasizes a need for the expansion of home health care. A 2021 Canadian survey reported 96% of seniors aged 65 and older prefer ageing in their own homes (National Institute on Ageing, 2021). With an aging population and increasingly long waitlists for long-term care homes, a shift to home care may be a promising solution for Canada's elder care crisis.

For those already living in nursing and long-term care homes, like Andrew, they received support in different ways than they were used to. Fiona mentioned that the homes would take them to bowling alleys, and groups of people visited them prior to the pandemic. She explained that their schedule remained busy with plenty of activities, though they were more on an individual level such as mental games or quizzes. In this particular case, Fiona recognizes the efforts made by the staff to keep them in the loop and maintain contact with their loved ones.

Of course, there is still much work that needs to be done to improve the health of seniors in long-term care homes. Currently, long-term care falls under provincial and territorial jurisdiction, and there has been a recent push for establishing national standards for long-term care homes (Jackson, 2021). Unlike most health services, the *Canada Health Act* does not define long-term care as a service that must be included by each provincial health insurance program in order to qualify for federal funds (Loprespub, 2020). Thus, a great proportion of long-term care homes are privately run. For example, in Ontario, 46% of long-term care homes are publicly owned, while 54% are privately owned (Loprespub, 2020). As a result, long-term care homes within provinces vary greatly in their standards and delivery of medical care. This gap in the regulation of long-term care homes has been brought to the attention of the federal government. In 2020, the federal government announced that it would work with the provinces and territories to establish national standards and that it would allocate $1 billion to implement infection control measures across long-term care homes (National Institute on Ageing, 2021). Hopefully, we can take the lessons learned from the past year to ensure our elderly population receives the protection they need from future outbreaks.

V. Persistence Through Teamwork, Patience, and Positivity

When asked for words of advice for the younger generation in regard to facing the pandemic and similar hardships in life, the interviewees all agreed on one theme: persistence. At first glance this may seem easier said than done, especially to younger people who are accustomed to immediate solutions. However, looking back at when the pandemic first broke out in the early spring of 2020, to where we are today, one can better appreciate the incredible endurance and strength we as a society have exhibited to fight through this battle. In the eyes of seniors, persistence is one of the most powerful tools that have helped them overcome challenges in life. They believe that persistence can be accomplished through three things: working as a team, being patient, and maintaining a positive outlook.

Because of how rapidly COVID-19 spreads through communities, teamwork is essential to protecting those around us. Recalling Eric's words, the elderly are one of the most at-risk populations in the face of COVID-19 due to their pre-existing health conditions, but this is something younger people often forget. As Emily saw younger individuals gathering in large groups, it is important for us to remember that our actions affect not only ourselves, but the entire community we live in. Sophie and Megan especially emphasized the importance of getting vaccinated and continuing to wear masks and follow social distancing measures.

They acknowledged the fatigue and restlessness younger people may be experiencing after over a year of restrictions, but emphasized that we must continue to endure and work together so we can end this pandemic sooner.

Many interviewees also noted that teamwork is an essential part of everyday life. Chris and Stephanie highlighted the importance of lending a hand to others in need, for tiny things like helping someone switch a lightbulb and bigger things like helping someone adjust to a new city. As individuals who have experienced the highs and lows of life, they understand that everyone is struggling with something, even if we can't see it on the outside. This has been especially key during the pandemic - no one has had it easy. Thus, we must learn to keep an open heart and embrace everyone like our own family.

With no foreseeable end to the pandemic in sight, many seniors also addressed the importance of patience. Michelle understands that youth are used to instantaneous solutions, due to the way they have grown up. The Internet is there for us when we need an answer to a question, and with text messages we can communicate with a friend within seconds. However, she urges younger people to be patient and live one day at a time. Similarly, Janet advises people to not get too bound on what is happening at the time and to remember that tomorrow is a new day, and Henry says drastic changes should be taken in stride. Only with patience will we be able to persist through the many challenges presented to us by the pandemic.

Lastly, many of the interviewees agreed that one of the most important elements to enduring the pandemic is positivity. Although sometimes we can't control what happens to us, what we can control is our attitude towards it. As Sean says, "live your life the best you can with what you're given." Knowing that there is a light at the end of the tunnel, we can spread positivity for a hopeful future and know that one day we will get to the other side. In Matilda's words, we must hang tight, stay optimistic, and assure ourselves that we can overcome this pandemic. In the meantime, embrace your loved ones, do the things you enjoy, and be kind to one another.

BIBLIOGRAPHY

Canadian Institute for Health Information. *Pandemic Experience in the Long-Term Care Sector: How Does Canada Compare With Other Countries?*. Ottawa, ON: CIHI; 2020.

Cheng, S., Zhao, Y., Kaminga, A. C., Zhang, P., & Xu, H. (2020). China's fight against COVID-19: What we have done and what we should do next? MedRxiv. https://doi.org/10.1101/2020.03.28.20046086

Coronavirus disease (COVID-19): Outbreak update. (2021, September 10). Government of Canada. https://www.canada.ca/en/public-health/services/diseases/2019-novel-coronavirus-infection.html?topic=tilelink

Cyranoski, D. (2020). What China's coronavirus response can teach the rest of the world. Nature, 579(7800), 479–480. https://doi.org/10.1038/d41586-020-00741-x

Devenyns, J. (2020, September 15). Consumers are eating at home more, but some are getting tired of it. Food Dive. https://www.fooddive.com/news/consumers-are-eating-at-home-more-but-some-are-getting-tired-of-it/585125/

Dong H. (2021). A Brief Summary of Pandemic Strategies in Wuhan. UWOMJ, 89(S1). Available from: https://ojs.lib.uwo.ca/index.php/uwomj/article/view/10658

Jackson, H. (2021, May 8). Establishing national standards for long-term care homes a 'huge priority': LeBlanc. Global News. https://globalnews.ca/news/7845375/leblanc-west-block-long-term-care-standards/

Koma, W., True, S., Biniek, J. F., Cubanski, J., Orgera, K., & Garfield, R. (2020, October 9). One in Four Older Adults Report Anxiety or Depression Amid the COVID-19 Pandemic. Kaiser Family Foundation. https://www.kff.org/medicare/issue-brief/one-in-four-older-adults-report-anxiety-or-depression-amid-the-covid-19-pandemic/

Loprespub. (2020, October 30). Long-Term Care Homes in Canada – How are They Funded and Regulated? HillNotes. https://hillnotes.ca/2020/10/22/long-term-care-homes-in-canada-how-are-they-funded-and-regulated/

Madan, A., Mrug, S., & Wright, R. A. (2013). The Effects of Media Violence on Anxiety in Late Adolescence. Journal of Youth and Adolescence, 43(1), 116–126. https://doi.org/10.1007/s10964-013-0017-3

National Institute on Ageing. (2021, March). Pandemic Perspectives on Long-Term Care: Insights from Canadians in Light of COVID-19. Canadian Medical Association.

Robertson, G. (2021, May 12). Pandemic errors made Canadian COVID-19 outbreak far worse than it needed to be, committee told. The Globe and Mail. https://www.theglobeandmail.com/canada/article-pandemic-errors-made-canadian-covid-19-outbreak-far-worse-than-it/

Smith, L. P., Ng, S. W., & Popkin, B. M. (2013). Trends in US home food preparation and consumption: analysis of national nutrition surveys and time use studies from 1965–1966 to 2007–2008. Nutrition Journal, 12(1). https://doi.org/10.1186/1475-2891-12-45

Staff. (2020, March 7). Coronavirus: Here's a timeline of COVID-19 cases in Canada. Global News. https://globalnews.ca/news/6627505/coronavirus-covid-canada-timeline/

Stern, A. M., Reilly, M. B., Cetron, M. S., & Markel, H. (2010). "Better off in School": School Medical Inspection as a Public Health Strategy during the 1918–1919 Influenza Pandemic in the United States. Public Health Reports, 125(3_suppl), 63–70. https://doi.org/10.1177/00333549101250s309

Vilches, T. N., Nourbakhsh, S., Zhang, K., Juden-Kelly, L., Cipriano, L. E., Langley, J. M., Sah, P., Galvani, A. P., & Moghadas, S. M. (2020). Multifaceted strategies for the control of COVID-19 outbreaks in long-term care facilities in Ontario, Canada. MedRxiv. https://doi.org/10.1101/2020.12.04.20244194

ACKNOWLEDGMENTS

There are several people we have to thank for making this book possible. First, we would like to thank all the seniors that we interviewed for taking the time to speak with us and for being as open as possible about sharing their personal life stories with the world. Secondly, we would like to thank Dr. Michel Lacerte for helping us recruit seniors, letting us use his office and equipment for our interviews, and his overall guidance on this book. We would also like to thank Stephanie for recruiting other seniors in her retirement residence. A big thanks to our fellow graduates from Western University, Disha Rawal for creating our cover art and Sebastian Deagle for helping with our initial stages of planning and creating our consent forms. We must not forget our editors Davis Dong, Sarah Verrault and Sana Zafar. Lastly, we would like to thank our family and friends for their support and encouragement during the creation of this book.

ABOUT THE AUTHORS

Viveka Sainani is a student at Western University, finishing an Honor Specialization in Medical Biophysics with a Minor in French. Her grandparents lived with her growing up and, through this, she grew an appreciation for their experience and advice. Through this book, she hopes to preserve their valuable voice and understand their perspective during the pandemic.

Shirley Liu is a first year master's student in the department of Medical Biophysics at Western University. She grew up with a love for writing short stories and novels. When the COVID-19 pandemic hit, she was motivated to combine her passion for storytelling with a desire to help communities make better informed policies surrounding care of the elderly population.

Nancy Liu is a first year medical student at the Schulich School of Medicine and Dentistry at Western University. She has a passion for community service and loves to learn about people's life stories. She hopes that through talking with others, she can gain a better understanding of the unmet needs of vulnerable populations and find ways to alleviate their struggles.

www.ingramcontent.com/pod-product-compliance
Lightning Source LLC
Chambersburg PA
CBHW030035230526
45472CB00002B/521